The Ultimate Keto Chaffle Diet Cookbook

Tasty and Affordable Breakfast Recipes to Start Your Day with the Right Foot

Kade Harrison

Table of Contents

Mini Breakfast Chaffles

Servings: 3
Cooking Time:
15 Minutes

Ingredients:

- 6 tsp coconut flour
- 1 tsp stevia
- 1/4 tsp baking powder
- 2 eggs
- 3 oz. cream cheese
- 1/2. tsp vanilla extract
- Topping
- 1 egg
- 6 slice bacon
- 2 oz. Raspberries for topping
- 2 oz. Blueberries for topping
- 2 oz. Strawberries for topping

Directions:

1. Heat up your square waffle maker and grease with cooking spray.
2. Mix together coconut flour, stevia, egg, baking powder, cheese and vanilla in mixing bowl.
3. Pour ½ of chaffles mixture in a waffle maker.
4. Close the lid and cook the chaffles for about 3-5 minutesutes.
5. Meanwhile, fry bacon slices in pan on medium heat for about 2-3 minutesutes until cooked and transfer themto plate.
6. In the same pan, fry eggs one by one in the leftover grease of bacon.

7. Once chaffles are cooked, carefully transferthem toplate.
8. Serve with fried eggs and bacon slice and berries on top.
9. Enjoy!

Nutrition: Protein: 16% 75 kcal Fat: 75% 346 kcal Carbohydrates: 9% 41 kcal

Crispy Chaffles With Egg & Asparagus

Servings:1

Cooking Time:

10 Minutes

Ingredients:

- 1 egg
- 1/4 cup cheddar cheese
- 2 tbsps. almond flour
- ½ tsp. baking powder
- TOPPING
- 1 egg
- 4-5 stalks asparagus
- 1 tsp avocado oil

Directions:

1. Preheat waffle maker to medium-high heat.
2. Whisk together egg, mozzarella cheese, almond flour, and baking powder
3. Pour chaffles mixture into the center of the waffle iron. Close the waffle maker and let cook for 5 minutesutes or until waffle is golden brown and set.
4. Remove chaffles from the waffle maker and serve.
5. Meanwhile, heat oil in a nonstick pan.
6. Once the pan is hot, fry asparagus for about 4-5 minutesutes until golden brown.
7. Poach the egg in boil water for about 2-3 minutesutes.
8. Once chaffles are cooked, remove from the maker.

9. Serve chaffles with the poached egg and asparagus.

Nutrition: Protein: 26% 85 kcal Fat: 69% 226 kcal Carbohydrates: 5% 16 kcal

Delicious Raspberries taco Chaffles

Servings:1

Cooking Time:

15 Minutes

Ingredients:

- 1 egg white
- 1/4 cup jack cheese, shredded
- 1/4 cup cheddar cheese, shredded
- 1 tsp coconut flour
- 1/4 tsp baking powder
- 1/2 tsp stevia
- For Topping
- 4 oz. raspberries
- 2 tbsps. coconut flour
- 2 oz. unsweetened raspberry sauce

Directions:

1. Switch on yourround Waffle Maker and grease it with cooking spray once it is hot.
2. Mix together all chaffle ingredients in a bowl and combine with a fork.
3. Pour chaffle batter in a preheated maker and close the lid.
4. Roll the taco chaffle around using a kitchen roller, set it aside and allow it to set for a few minutesutes.
5. Once the taco chaffle is set, remove from the roller.
6. Dip raspberries in sauce and arrange on taco chaffle.
7. Drizzle coconut flour on top.
8. Enjoy raspberries taco chaffle with keto coffee.

Nutrition: Protein: 28% 77 kcal Fat: 6 187 kcal
Carbohydrates: 3% 8 kcal

Coconut Chaffles

Servings: 2
Cooking Time:
5 Minutes

Ingredients:

- 1 egg
- 1 oz. cream cheese,
- 1 oz. cheddar cheese
- 2 tbsps. coconut flour
- 1 tsp. stevia
- 1 tbsp. coconut oil, melted
- 1/2 tsp. coconut extract
- 2 eggs, soft boil for serving

Directions:

1. Heat you minutes Dash waffle maker and grease with cooking spray.
2. Mix together all chaffles ingredients in a bowl.
3. Pour chaffle batter in a preheated waffle maker.
4. Close the lid.
5. Cook chaffles for about 2-3 minutes until golden brown.
6. Serve with boil egg and enjoy!

Nutrition: Protein: 21% 32 kcal Fat: % 117 kcal
Carbohydrates: 3% 4 kcal

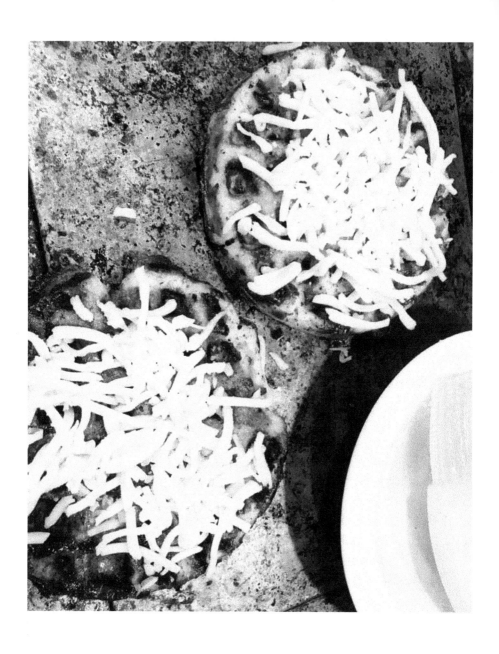

Garlic And Parsley Chaffles

Servings:1

Cooking Time:

5 Minutes

Ingredients:

- 1 large egg
- 1/4 cup cheese mozzarella
- 1 tsp. coconut flour
- ¼ tsp. baking powder
- ½ tsp. garlic powder
- 1 tbsp. minutesced parsley
- For Serving
- 1 Poach egg
- 4 oz. smoked salmon

Directions:

1. Switch on your Dash minutes waffle maker and let it preheat.
2. Grease waffle maker with cooking spray.
3. Mix together egg, mozzarella, coconut flour, baking powder, and garlic powder, parsley to a mixing bowl until combined well.
4. Pour batter in circle chaffle maker.
5. Close the lid.
6. Cook for about 2-3 minutes or until the chaffles are cooked.
7. Serve with smoked salmon and poached egg.
8. Enjoy!

Nutrition: Protein: 45% 140 kcal Fat: 51% 160 kcal
Carbohydrates: 4% 14 kcal

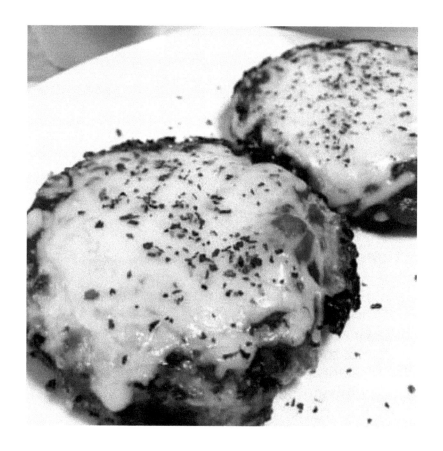

Scrambled Eggs On A Spring Onion Chaffle

Servings:4

Cooking Time:

7–9 Minutes

Ingredients:

- Batter
- 4 eggs
- 2 cups grated mozzarella cheese
- 2 spring onions, finely chopped
- Salt and pepper to taste
- ½ teaspoon dried garlic powder
- 2 tablespoons almond flour
- 2 tablespoons coconut flour
- Other
- 2 tablespoons butter for brushing the waffle maker
- 6-8 eggs
- Salt and pepper
- 1 teaspoon Italian spice mix
- 1 tablespoon olive oil
- 1 tablespoon freshly chopped parsley

Directions:

1. Preheat the waffle maker.
2. Crack the eggs into a bowl and add the grated cheese.
3. Mix until just combined, then add the chopped spring onions and season with salt and pepper and dried garlic powder.

4. Stir in the almond flour and mix until everything is combined.
5. Brush the heated waffle maker with butter and add a few tablespoons of the batter.
6. Close the lid and cook for about 7–8 minutes depending on your waffle maker.
7. While the chaffles are cooking, prepare the scrambled eggs by whisking the eggs in a bowl until frothy, about 2 minutes. Season with salt and black pepper to taste and add the Italian spice mix. Whisk to blend in the spices.
8. Warm the oil in a non-stick pan over medium heat.
9. Pour the eggs in the pan and cook until eggs are set to your liking.
10. Serve each chaffle and top with some scrambled eggs. Top with freshly chopped parsley.

Nutrition: Calories: 194, Fat: 14.7 g, Carbs: 5 g, Sugar: 0.6 g, Protein: 1 g, Sodium: 191 mg

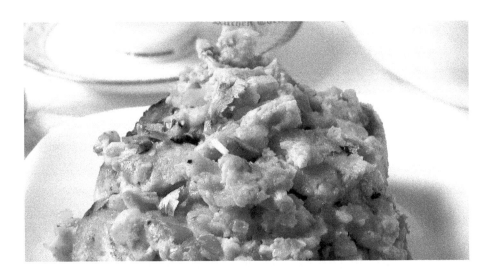

Egg On A Cheddar Cheese Chaffle

Servings:4

Cooking Time:

7–9 Minutes

Ingredients:

- Batter
- 4 eggs
- 2 cups shredded white cheddar cheese
- Salt and pepper to taste
- Other
- 2 tablespoons butter for brushing the waffle maker
- 4 large eggs
- 2 tablespoons olive oil

Directions:

1. Preheat the waffle maker.
2. Crack the eggs into a bowl and whisk them with a fork.
3. Stir in the grated cheddar cheese and season with salt and pepper.
4. Brush the heated waffle maker with butter and add a few tablespoons of the batter.
5. Close the lid and cook for about 7–8 minutes depending on your waffle maker.
6. While chaffles are cooking, cook the eggs.
7. Warm the oil in a large non-stick pan that has a lid over medium-low heat for 2-3 minutes
8. Crack an egg in a small ramekin and gently add it to the pan. Repeat the same way for the other 3 eggs.

9. Cover and let cook for 2 to 2 ½ minutes for set eggs but with runny yolks.
10.   Remove from heat.
11.   To serve, place a chaffle on each plate and top with an egg. Season with salt and black pepper to taste.

Nutrition: Calories 4 fat 34 g, carbs 2 g, sugar 0.6 g, Protein 26 g, sodium 518 mg

Avocado Chaffle Toast

Servings:3

Cooking Time:

10 Minutes

Ingredients:

- 4 tbsps. avocado mash
- 1/2 tsp lemon juice
- 1/8 tsp salt
- 1/8 tsp black pepper
- 2 eggs
- 1/2 cup shredded cheese
- For serving
- 3 eggs
- ½ avocado thinly sliced
- 1 tomato, sliced

Directions:

1. Mash avocado mash with lemon juice, salt, and black pepper in mixing bowl, until well combined.
2. In a small bowl beat egg and pour eggs in avocado mixture and mix well.
3. Switch on Waffle Maker to pre-heat.
4. Pour 1/8 of shredded cheese in a waffle maker and then pour ½ of egg and avocado mixture and then 1/8 shredded cheese.
5. Close the lid and cook chaffles for about 3 - 4 minutesutes.
6. Repeat with the remaining mixture.
7. Meanwhile,fry eggs in a pan for about 1-2 minutesutes.

8. For serving, arrange fried egg on chaffle toast with avocado slice and tomatoes.
9. Sprinkle salt and pepper on top and enjoy!

Nutrition: Protein: 26% 66 kcal Fat: 67% 169 kcal Carbohydrates: 6% 15 kcal

Cajun & Feta Chaffles

Servings:1

Cooking Time:

10 Minutes

Ingredients:

- 1 egg white
- 1/4 cup shredded mozzarella cheese
- 2 tbsps. almond flour
- 1 tsp Cajun Seasoning
- FOR SERVING
- 1 egg
- 4 oz. feta cheese
- 1 tomato, sliced

Directions:

1. Whisk together egg, cheese, and seasoning in a bowl.
2. Switch on and grease waffle maker with cooking spray.
3. Pour batter in a preheated waffle maker.
4. Cook chaffles for about 2-3 minutesutes until the chaffle is cooked through.
5. Meanwhile, fry the egg in a non-stick pan for about 1-2 minutesutes.
6. For serving set fried egg on chaffles with feta cheese and tomatoes slice.

Nutrition: Protein: 28% 119 kcal Fat: 64% 2 kcal Carbohydrates: 7% 31 kcal

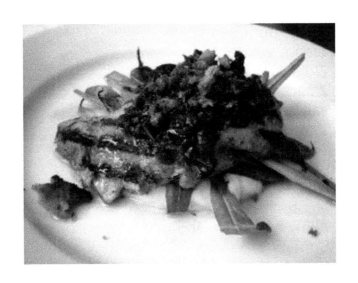

Crispy Chaffles With Sausage

Servings: 2

Cooking Time:

10 Minutes

Ingredients:

- 1/2 cup cheddar cheese
- 1/2 tsp. baking powder
- 1/4 cup egg whites
- 2 tsp. pumpkin spice
- 1 egg, whole
- 2 chicken sausage
- 2 slice bacon
- salt and pepper to taste
- 1 tsp. avocado oil

Directions:

1. Mix together all ingredients in a bowl.
2. Allow batter to sit while waffle iron warms.
3. Spray waffle iron with nonstick spray.
4. Pour batter in the waffle maker and cook according to the directions of the manufacturer.
5. Meanwhile, heat oil in a pan and fry the egg, according to your choice and transfer it toa plate.
6. In the same pan, fry bacon slice and sausage on medium heat for about 2-3 minutesutes until cooked.
7. Once chaffles are cooked thoroughly, remove them from the maker.
8. Serve with fried egg, bacon slice, sausages and enjoy!

Nutrition: Protein: 22% 86 kcal Fat: 74% 286 kcal
Carbohydrates: 3% 12 kcal

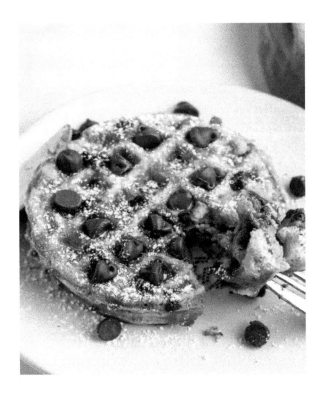

Chili Chaffle

Servings: 4

Cooking Time:
7–9 Minutes

Ingredients:

- Batter
- 4 eggs
- ½ cup grated parmesan cheese
- 1½ cups grated yellow cheddar cheese
- 1 hot red chili pepper
- Salt and pepper to taste
- ½ teaspoon dried garlic powder
- 1 teaspoon dried basil
- 2 tablespoons almond flour
- Other
- 2 tablespoons olive oil for brushing the waffle maker

Directions:

1. Preheat the waffle maker.
2. Crack the eggs into a bowl and add the grated parmesan and cheddar cheese.
3. Mix until just combined and add the chopped chili pepper. Season with salt and pepper, dried garlic powder and dried basil.
4. Stir in the almond flour.
5. Mix until everything is combined.
6. Brush the heated waffle maker with olive oil and add a few tablespoons of the batter.
7. Close the lid and cook for about 7–8 minutes depending on your waffle maker.

Nutrition: Calories 36 fat 30.4 g, carbs 3.1 g, sugar 0.7 g, Protein 21.5 g, sodium 469 mg

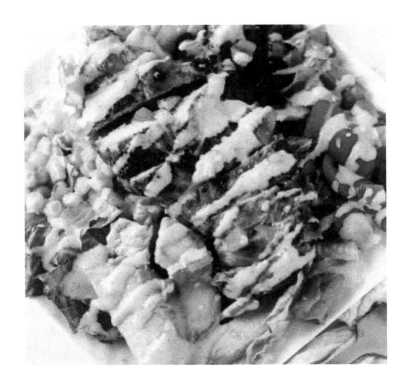

Simple Savory Chaffle

Servings:4

Cooking Time:

7–9 Minutes

Ingredients:

- Batter
- 4 eggs
- 1 cup grated mozzarella cheese
- 1 cup grated provolone cheese
- ½ cup almond flour
- 2 tablespoons coconut flour
- 2½ teaspoons baking powder
- Salt and pepper to taste
- Other
- 2 tablespoons butter to brush the waffle maker

Directions:

1. Preheat the waffle maker.
2. Add the grated mozzarella and provolone cheese to a bowl and mix.
3. Add the almond and coconut flour and baking powder and season with salt and pepper.
4. Mix with a wire whisk and crack in the eggs.
5. Stir everything together until batter forms.
6. Brush the heated waffle maker with butter and add a few tablespoons of the batter.
7. Close the lid and cook for about 8 minutes depending on your waffle maker.
8. Serve and enjoy.

Nutrition: Calories 352, fat 27.2 g, carbs 8.3 g, sugar 0.5 g, Protein 15 g, sodium 442 mg

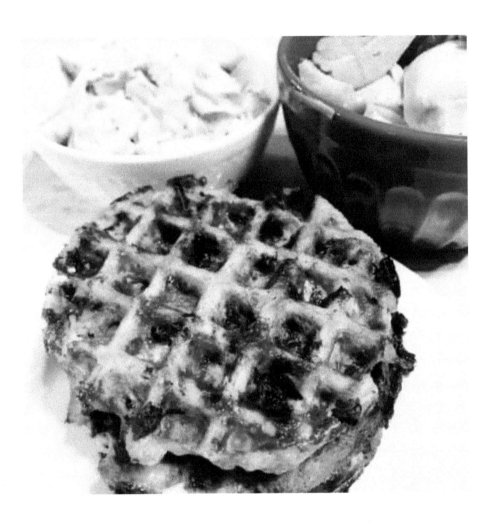

Pizza Chaffle

Servings: 4

Cooking Time:

7–9 Minutes

Ingredients:

- Batter
- 4 eggs
- 1½ cups grated mozzarella cheese
- ½ cup grated parmesan cheese
- 2 tablespoons tomato sauce
- ¼ cup almond flour
- 1½ teaspoons baking powder
- Salt and pepper to taste
- 1 teaspoon dried oregano
- ¼ cup sliced salami
- Other
- 2 tablespoons olive oil for brushing the waffle maker
- ¼ cup tomato sauce for serving

Directions:

1. Preheat the waffle maker.
2. Add the grated mozzarella and grated parmesan to a bowl and mix.
3. Add the almond flour and baking powder and season with salt and pepper and dried oregano.
4. Mix with a wooden spoon or wire whisk and crack in the eggs.
5. Stir everything together until batter forms.
6. Stir in the chopped salami.

7. Brush the heated waffle maker with olive oil and add a few tablespoons of the batter.
8. Close the lid and cook for about 7–minutes depending on your waffle maker.
9. Serve with extra tomato sauce on top and enjoy.

Nutrition: Calories 319, fat 25.2 g, carbs 5.9 g, sugar 1.7 g, Protein 19.3 g, sodium 596 mg

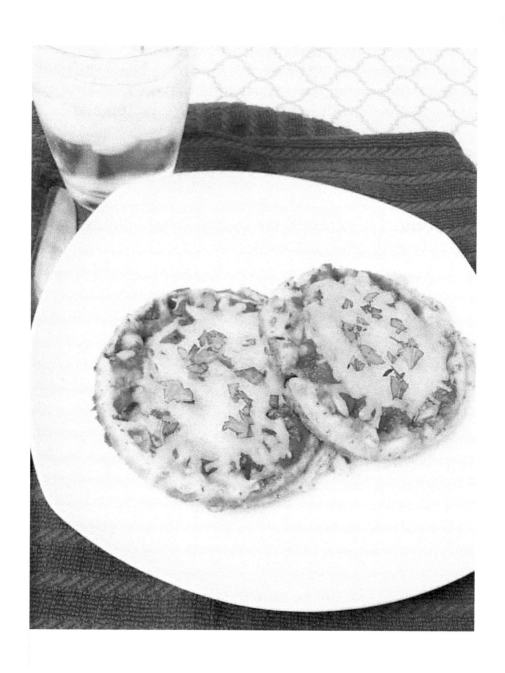

Bacon Chaffle

Servings:4
Cooking Time:
7–9 Minutes

Ingredients:

- Batter
- 4 eggs
- 2 cups shredded mozzarella
- 2 ounces finely chopped bacon
- Salt and pepper to taste
- 1 teaspoon dried oregano
- Other
- 2 tablespoons olive oil for brushing the waffle maker

Directions:

1. Preheat the waffle maker.
2. Crack the eggs into a bowl and add the grated mozzarella cheese.
3. Mix until just combined and stir in the chopped bacon.
4. Season with salt and pepper and dried oregano.
5. Brush the heated waffle maker with olive oil and add a few tablespoons of the batter.
6. Close the lid and cook for about 7–8 minutes depending on your waffle maker.

Nutrition: Calories 241, fat 19.8 g, carbs 1.3 g, sugar 0.4 g, Protein 14.8 g, sodium 4 mg

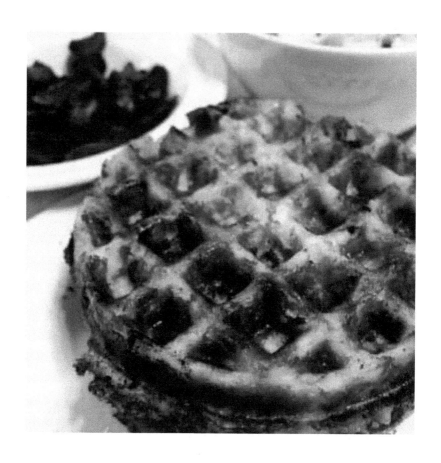

Chaffles Breakfast Bowl

Servings:2

Cooking Time:

5 Minutes

Ingredients:

- 1 egg
- 1/2 cup cheddar cheese shredded
- pinch of Italian seasoning
- 1 tbsp. pizza sauce
- TOPPING
- 1/2 avocado sliced
- 2 eggs boiled
- 1 tomato, halves
- 4 oz. fresh spinach leaves

Directions:

1. Preheat your waffle maker and grease with cooking spray.
2. Crack an egg in a small bowl and beat with Italian seasoning and pizza sauce.
3. Add shredded cheese to the egg and spices mixture.
4. Pour 1 tbsp. shredded cheese in a waffle maker and cook for 30 sec.
5. Pour Chaffles batter inthe waffle maker and close the lid.
6. Cook chaffles for about 4 minutesutes until crispy and brown.Carefully remove chaffles from the maker.
7. Serve on the bed of spinach with boil egg, avocado slice, and tomatoes.
8. Enjoy!!

Nutrition: Protein: 23% 77 kcal Fat: 66% 222 kcal Carbohydrates: 11% 39 kcal

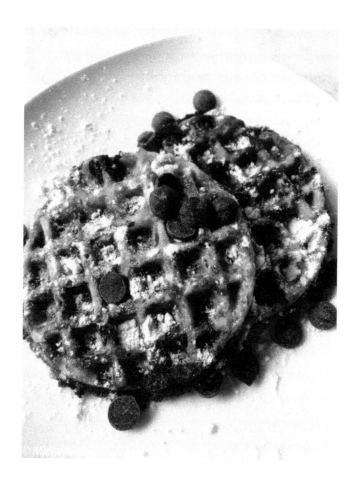

Morning Chaffles With Berries

Servings: 4

Cooking Time:

5 Minutes

Ingredients:

- 1 cup egg whites
- 1 cup cheddar cheese, shredded
- ¼ cup almond flour
- ¼ cup heavy cream
- TOPPING
- 4 oz. raspberries
- 4 oz. strawberries.
- 1 oz. keto chocolate flakes
- 1 oz. feta cheese.

Directions:

1. Preheat your square waffle maker and grease with cooking spray.
2. Beat egg white in a small bowl with flour.
3. Add shredded cheese to the egg whites and flour mixture and mix well.
4. Add cream and cheese tothe egg mixture.
5. Pour Chaffles batter in a waffle maker and close the lid.
6. Cook chaffles for about 4 minutesutes until crispy and brown.
7. Carefully remove chaffles from the maker.
8. Serve with berries, cheese, and chocolate on top.
9. Enjoy!

Nutrition: Protein: 28% 68 kcal Fat: 67% 163 kcal
Carbohydrates: 5% 12 kcal

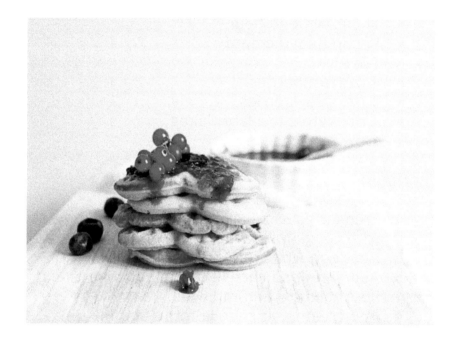

Chicken Bites With Chaffles

Servings: 2

Cooking Time:

10 minutes

Ingredients:

- 1 chicken breast cut into 2 x2 inch chunks
- 1 egg, whisked
- 1/4 cup almond flour
- 2 tbsps. onion powder
- 2 tbsps. garlic powder
- 1 tsp. dried oregano
- 1 tsp. paprika powder
- 1 tsp. salt
- 1/2 tsp. black pepper
- 2 tbsps. avocado oil

Directions:

1. Add all the dry ingredients together into a large bowl.
2. Mix well.
3. Place the eggs into a separate bowl.
4. Dip each chicken piece into the egg and then into the dry ingredients.
5. Heat oil in 10-inch skillet, add oil.
6. Once avocado oil is hot, place the coated chicken nuggets onto a skillet and cook for 6-8 minutesutes until cooked and golden brown.
7. Serve with chaffles and raspberries.
8. Enjoy!

Nutrition: Total Calories: 401 kcal Fats: 219 g Protein: 32.35 g Carbs: 1.46 g Fiber: 3 g

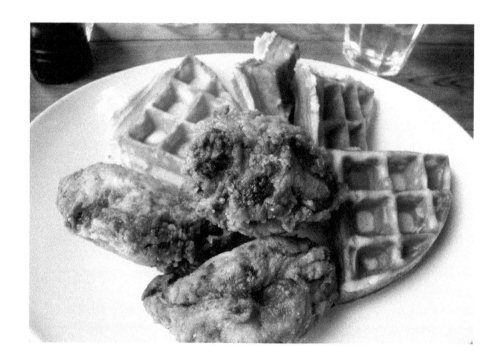

Crunchy Fish And Waffle Bites

Servings:4

Cooking Time:

15 Minutes

Ingredients:

- 1 lb. cod fillets, sliced into 4 slice
- 1 tsp. sea salt
- 1 tsp. garlic powder
- 1 egg, whisked
- 1 cup almond flour
- 2 tbsp. avocado oil
- CHAFFLE Ingredients:
- 2 eggs
- 1/2 cup cheddar cheese
- 2 tbsps. almond flour
- ½ tsp. Italian seasoning

Directions:

1. Mix together chaffle ingredients in a bowl and make 4 square
2. Put the chaffles in a preheated chaffle maker.
3. Mix together the salt, pepper, and garlic powder in a mixing bowl. Toss the cod cubes in this mixture and let sit for 10 minutesutes.
4. Then dip each cod slice into the egg mixture and then into the almond flour.
5. Heat oil in skillet and fish cubes for about 2-3 minutesutes, until cooked and browned
6. Serve on chaffles and enjoy!

Nutrition: Protein: 38% 121 kcal Fat: 59% 189 kcal
Carbohydrates: 3% 11 kcal

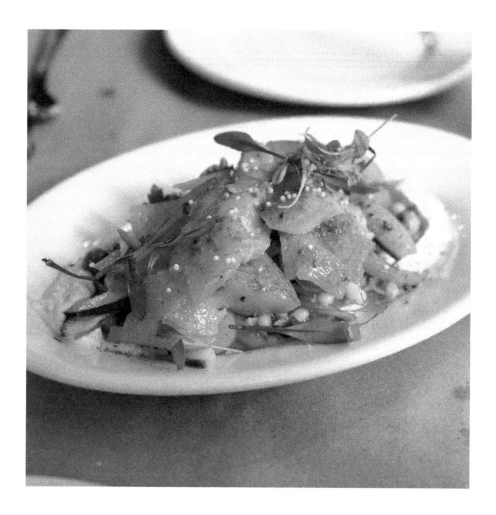

Grill Pork Chaffle Sandwich

Servings:2
Cooking Time:
15 Minutes

Ingredients:

- 1/2 cup mozzarella, shredded
- 1 egg
- I pinch garlic powder
- PORK PATTY
- 1/2 cup pork, minutesced
- 1 tbsp. green onion, diced
- 1/2 tsp Italian seasoning
- Lettuce leaves

Directions:

1. Preheat the square waffle maker and grease with
2. Mix together egg, cheese and garlic powder in a small mixing bowl.
3. Pour batter in a preheated waffle maker and close the lid.
4. Make 2 chaffles from thisbatter.
5. Cook chaffles for about 2-3 minutesutes until cooked through.
6. Meanwhile, mix together pork patty ingredients in a bowl and make 1 large patty.
7. Grill pork patty in a preheated grill for about 3-4 minutesutes per side until cooked through.
8. Arrange pork patty between two chaffles with lettuce leaves. Cut sandwich to make a triangular sandwich.

9. Enjoy!

Nutrition: Protein: 48% 85 kcal Fat: 48% 86 kcal
Carbohydrates: 4% 7 kcal

Chaffle & Chicken Lunch Plate

Servings:1
Cooking Time:
15 Minutes

Ingredients:

- 1 large egg
- 1/2 cup jack cheese, shredded
- 1 pinch salt
- For Serving
- 1 chicken leg
- salt
- pepper
- 1 tsp. garlic, minutesced
- 1 egg
- I tsp avocado oil

Directions:

1. Heat your square waffle maker and grease with cooking spray.
2. Pour Chaffle batter intothe skillet and cook for about 3 minutesutes.
3. Meanwhile,heat oil in a pan, over medium heat.
4. Once the oil is hot, add chicken thigh and garlicthen, cook for about 5 minutesutes. Flip and cook for another 3-4 minutesutes.
5. Season with salt and pepper and give them a good mix.
6. Transfer cooked thigh to plate.
7. Fry the egg in the same pan for about 1-2 minutesutes according to your choice.

8. Once chaffles are cooked, serve with fried egg and chicken thigh.
9. Enjoy!

Nutrition: Protein: 31% 138 kcal Fat: 66% 292 kcal Carbohydrates: 2% kcal

Chaffle Egg Sandwich

Servings: 2

Cooking Time:

10 Minutes

Ingredients:

- 2 minutesI keto chaffle
- 2 slice cheddar cheese
- 1 egg simple omelet

Directions:

1. Prepare your oven on 4000 F.
2. Arrange egg omelet and cheese slice between chaffles.
3. Bake in the preheated oven for about 4-5 minutesutes until cheese is melted.
4. Once the cheese is melted, remove from the oven.
5. Serve and enjoy!

Nutrition: Protein: 29% 144 kcal Fat: % 337 kcal Carbohydrates: 3% 14 kcal

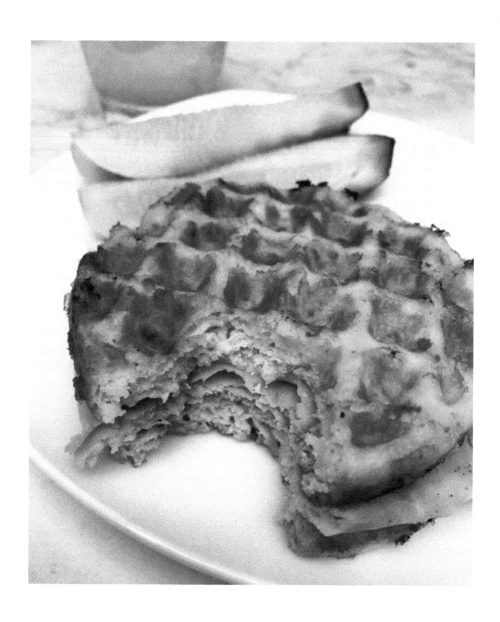

Chaffle Minutesi Sandwich

Servings: 2

Cooking Time:

10 Minutes

Ingredients:

- 1 large egg
- 1/8 cup almond flour
- 1/2 tsp. garlic powder
- 3/4 tsp. baking powder
- 1/2 cup shredded cheese
- SANDWICH FILLING
- 2 slices deli ham
- 2 slices tomatoes
- 1 slice cheddar cheese

Directions:

1. Grease your square waffle maker and preheat it on medium heat.
2. Mix together chaffle ingredients in a mixing bowl until well combined.
3. Pour batter intoa square waffle and make two chaffles.
4. Once chaffles are cooked, remove from the maker.
5. For a sandwich,arrange deli ham, tomato slice and cheddar cheese between two chaffles.
6. Cut sandwich from the center.
7. Serve and enjoy!

Nutrition: Protein: 29% 70 kcal Fat: 66% 159 kcal
Carbohydrates: 4% 10 kcal

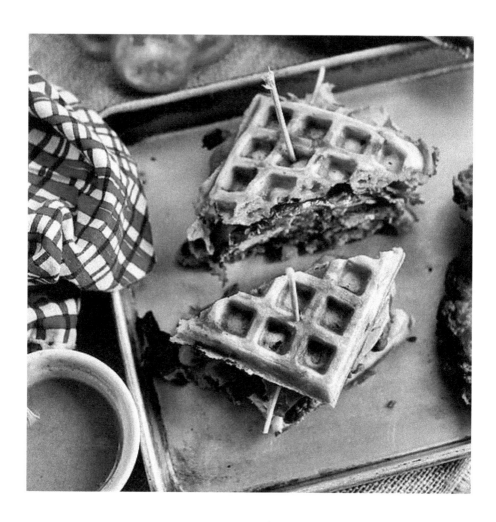

Chaffle Cheese Sandwich

Servings: 1

Cooking Time:

10 Minutes

Ingredients:

- 2 square keto chaffle
- 2 slice cheddar cheese
- 2 lettuce leaves

Directions:

1. Prepare your oven on 4000 F.
2. Arrange lettuce leave and cheese slice between chaffles.
3. Bake in the preheated oven for about 4-5 minutesutes until cheese is melted.
4. Once the cheese is melted, remove from the oven.
5. Serve and enjoy!

Nutrition: Protein: 28% kcal Fat: 69% 149 kcal Carbohydrates: 3% 6 kcal

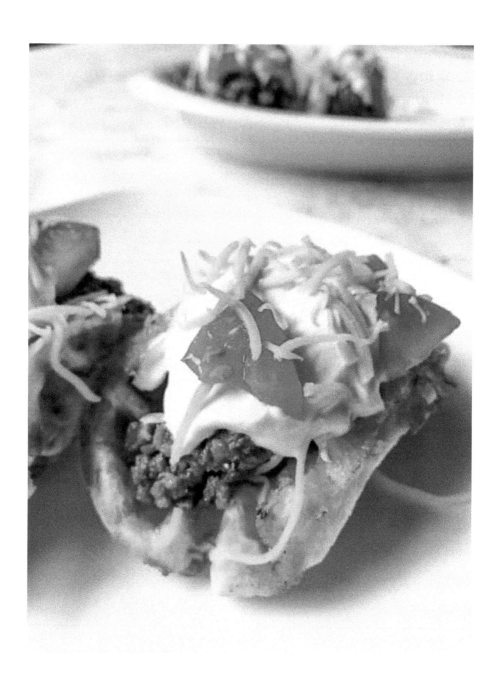

Chicken Zinger Chaffle

Servings:2

Cooking Time:

15 Minutes

Ingredients:

- 1 chicken breast, cut into 2 pieces
- 1/2 cup coconut flour
- 1/4 cup finely grated Parmesan
- 1 tsp. paprika
- 1/2 tsp. garlic powder
- 1/2 tsp. onion powder
- 1 tsp. salt& pepper
- 1 egg beaten
- Avocado oil for frying
- Lettuce leaves
- BBQ sauce
- CHAFFLE Ingredients:
- 4 oz. cheese
- 2 whole eggs
- 2 oz. almond flour
- 1/4 cup almond flour
- 1 tsp baking powder

Directions:

1. Mix together chaffle ingredients in a bowl.
2. Pour the chaffle batter in preheated greased square chaffle maker.
3. Cook chaffles for about 2-minutesutes until cooked through.
4. Make square chaffles from this batter.

5. Meanwhile mix together coconut flour, parmesan, paprika, garlic powder, onion powder salt and pepper in a bowl.
6. Dip chicken first in coconut flour mixture then in beaten egg.
7. Heat avocado oil in a skillet and cook chicken from both sides. until lightly brown and cooked
8. Set chicken zinger between two chaffles with lettuce and BBQ sauce.
9. Enjoy!

Nutrition: Protein: 30% 219 kcal Fat: 60% 435 kcal Carbohydrates: 9% 66 kcal

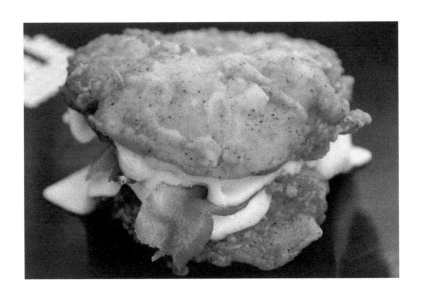

Double Chicken Chaffles

Servings:2
Cooking Time:
5 Minutes

Ingredients:

- 1/2 cup boil shredded chicken
- 1/4 cup cheddar cheese
- 1/8 cup parmesan cheese
- 1 egg
- 1 tsp. Italian seasoning
- 1/8 tsp. garlic powder
- 1 tsp. cream cheese

Directions:

1. Preheat the Belgian waffle maker.
2. Mix together in chaffle ingredients in a bowl and mix together.
3. Sprinkle 1 tbsp. of cheese in a waffle maker and pour in chaffle batter.
4. Pour 1 tbsp. of cheese over batter and close the lid.
5. Cook chaffles for about 4 to minutesutes.
6. Serve with a chicken zinger and enjoy the double chicken flavor.

Nutrition: Protein: 30% 60 kcal Fat: 65% 129 kcal Carbohydrates: 5% 9 kcal

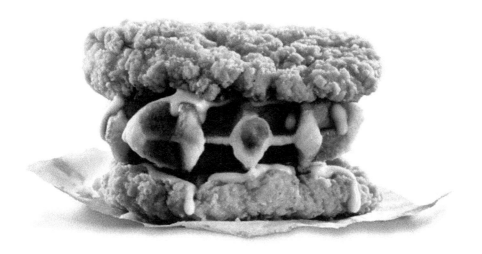

Chaffles With Topping

Servings: 3

Cooking Time:

10 Minutes

Ingredients:

- 1 large egg
- 1 tbsp. almond flour
- 1 tbsp. full-fat Greek yogurt
- 1/8 tsp baking powder
- 1/4 cup shredded Swiss cheese
- TOPPING
- 4oz. grillprawns
- 4 oz. steamed cauliflower mash
- 1/2 zucchini sliced
- 3 lettuce leaves
- 1 tomato, sliced
- 1 tbsp. flax seeds

Directions:

1. Make 3 chaffles with the given chaffles ingredients.
2. For serving, arrange lettuce leaves on each chaffle.
3. Top with zucchini slice, grill prawns, cauliflower mash and a tomato slice.
4. Drizzle flax seeds on top.
5. Serve and enjoy!

Nutrition: Protein: 45% 71 kcal Fat: 47% 75 kcal
Carbohydrates: 8% 12 kcal

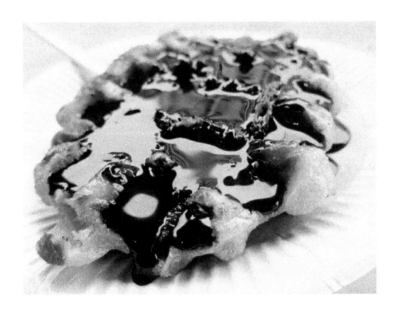

Chaffle With Cheese & Bacon

Servings:2

Cooking Time:

15 Minutes

Ingredients:

- 1 egg
- 1/2 cup cheddar cheese, shredded
- 1 tbsp. parmesan cheese
- 3/4 tsp coconut flour
- 1/4 tsp baking powder
- 1/8 tsp Italian Seasoning
- pinch of salt
- 1/4 tsp garlic powder
- FOR TOPPING
- 1 bacon sliced, cooked and chopped
- 1/2 cup mozzarella cheese, shredded
- 1/4 tsp parsley, chopped

Directions:

1. Preheat oven to 400 degrees.
2. Switch on your minutesi waffle maker and grease with cooking spray.
3. Mix together chaffle ingredients in a mixing bowl until combined.
4. Spoon half of the batter in the center of the waffle maker and close the lid. Cook chaffles for about 3-minutesutes until cooked.
5. Carefully remove chaffles from the maker.
6. Arrange chaffles in a greased baking tray.
7. Top with mozzarella cheese, chopped bacon and parsley.
8. And bake in the oven for 4 -5 minutesutes.

9. Once the cheese is melted, remove from the oven.
10.   Serve and enjoy!

Nutrition: Protein: 28% 90 kcal Fat: 69% 222 kcal Carbohydrates: 3% kcal

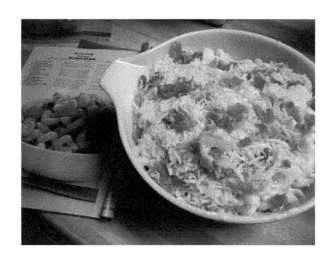

Grill Beefsteak And Chaffle

Servings: 1

Cooking Time:

10 Minutes

Ingredients:

- 1 beefsteak rib eye
- 1 tsp salt
- 1 tsp pepper
- 1 tbsp. lime juice
- 1 tsp garlic

Directions:

1. Prepare your grill for direct heat.
2. Mix together all spices and rub over beefsteak evenly.
3. Place the beef on the grill rack over medium heat.
4. Cover and cook steak for about6 to 8 minutesutes. Flip and cook for another 5 minutesutes until cooked through.
5. Serve with keto simple chaffle and enjoy!

Nutrition: Protein: 51% 274 kcal Fat: 45% 243 kcal Carbohydrates: 4% 22 kcal

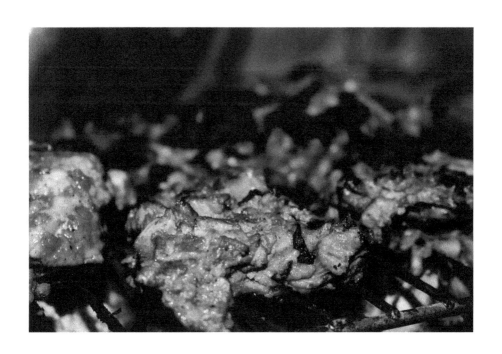

Cauliflower Chaffles And Tomatoes

Servings:2

Cooking Time:

15 Minutes

Ingredients:

- 1/2 cup cauliflower
- 1/4 tsp. garlic powder
- 1/4 tsp. black pepper
- 1/4 tsp. Salt
- 1/2 cup shredded cheddar cheese
- 1 egg
- FOR TOPPING
- 1 lettuce leave
- 1 tomato sliced
- 4 oz. cauliflower steamed, mashed
- 1 tsp sesame seeds

Directions:

1. Add all chaffle ingredients into a blender and mix well.
2. Sprinkle 1/8 shredded cheese on the waffle maker and pour cauliflower mixture in a preheated waffle maker and sprinkle the rest of the cheese over it.
3. Cook chaffles for about 4-5 minutesutes until cooked
4. For serving, lay lettuce leaves over chaffle top with steamed cauliflower and tomato.
5. Drizzle sesame seeds on top.
6. Enjoy!

Nutrition: Protein: 25% 49 kcal Fat: 65% 128 kcal
Carbohydrates: 10% 21 kcal

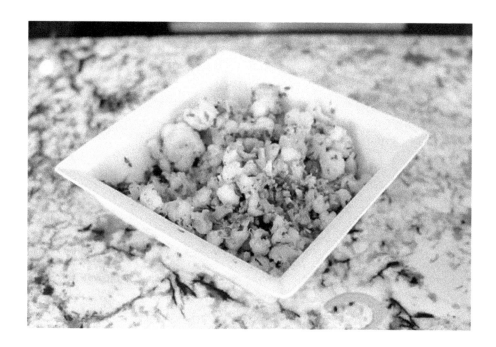

Layered Cheese Chaffles

Servings: 1
Cooking Time:
5 Minutes

Ingredients:

- 1 organic egg, beaten
- 1/3 cup Cheddar cheese, shredded
- ½ teaspoon ground flaxseed
- ¼ teaspoon organic baking powder
- 2 tablespoons Parmesan cheese, shredded

Directions:

1. Preheat a mini waffle iron and then grease it.
2. In a bowl, place all the ingredients except Parmesan and beat until well combined.
3. Place half the Parmesan cheese in the bottom of preheated waffle iron.
4. Place half of the egg mixture over cheese and top with the remaining Parmesan cheese.
5. Cook for about 3-minutes or until golden brown.
6. Serve warm.

Nutrition: Calories: 264 Carb: 1 Fat: 20g Saturated Fat: 11.1 g Carbohydrates: 2.1g Dietary Fiber: 0.4g Sugar: 0.6g Protein: 18.9g

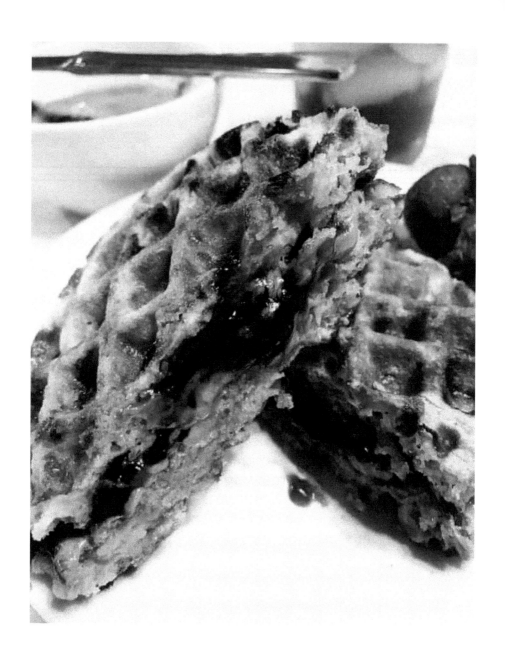

Chaffles With Keto Ice Cream

Servings: 2

Cooking Time:

14 Minutes

Ingredients:

- 1 egg, beaten
- ½ cup finely grated mozzarella cheese
- ¼ cup almond flour
- 2 tbsp swerve confectioner's sugar
- 1/8 tsp xanthan gum
- Low-carb ice cream (flavor of your choice) for serving

Directions:

1. Preheat the waffle iron.
2. In a medium bowl, mix all the ingredients except the ice cream.
3. Open the iron and add half of the mixture. Close and cook until crispy, 7 minutes.
4. Transfer the chaffle to a plate and make second one with the remaining batter.
5. On each chaffle, add a scoop of low carb ice cream, fold into half-moons and enjoy.

Nutrition: Calories: 89 Fat: 48g Carbs: 1.67g Protein: 5.91g

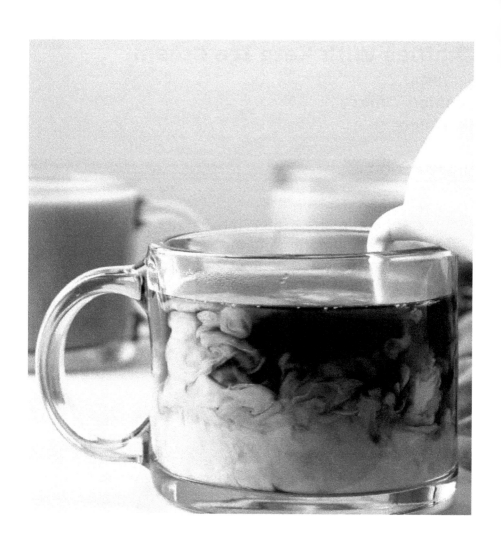

Vanilla Mozzarella Chaffles

Servings: 2

Cooking Time:

12 Minutes

Ingredients:

- 1 organic egg, beaten
- 1 teaspoon organic vanilla extract
- 1 tablespoon almond flour
- 1 teaspoon organic baking powder
- Pinch of ground cinnamon
- 1 cup Mozzarella cheese, shredded

Directions:

1. Preheat a mini waffle iron and then grease it.
2. In a bowl, place the egg and vanilla extract and beat until well combined.
3. Add the flour, baking powder and cinnamon and mix well.
4. Add the Mozzarella cheese and stir to combine.
5. In a small bowl, place the egg and Mozzarella cheese and stir to combine.
6. Place half of the mixture into preheated waffle iron and cook for about 5-minutes or until golden brown.
7. Repeat with the remaining mixture.
8. Serve warm.

Nutrition: Calories: 103 Carb: 2.4g Fat: 6.6g Saturated Fat: 2.3g Carbohydrates: 2 Dietary Fiber: 0.5g Sugar: 0.6g Protein: 6.8g

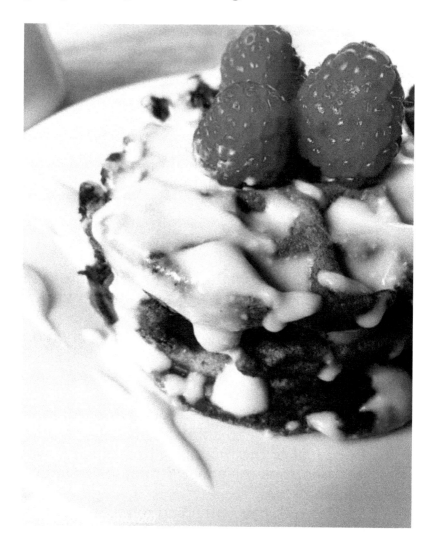

Bruschetta Chaffle

Servings: 2

Cooking Time:

5 Minutes

Ingredients:

- 2 basic chaffles
- 2 tablespoons sugar-free marinara sauce
- 2 tablespoons mozzarella, shredded
- 1 tablespoon olives, sliced
- 1 tomato sliced
- 1 tablespoon keto friendly pesto sauce
- Basil leaves

Directions:

1. Spread marinara sauce on each chaffle.
2. Spoon pesto and spread on top of the marinara sauce.
3. Top with the tomato, olives and mozzarella.
4. Bake in the oven for 3 minutes or until the cheese has melted.
5. Garnish with basil.
6. Serve and enjoy.

Nutrition: Calories: 182 Total Fat: 11g Saturated Fat: 6.1g Cholesterol: 30mg Sodium: 508mg Potassium: 1mg Total Carbohydrate: 3.1 g Dietary Fiber: 1.1g Protein: 16.8g Total Sugars: 1g

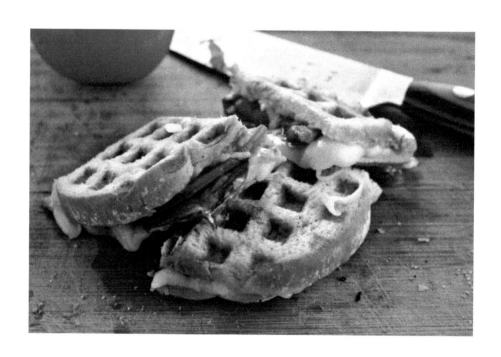

Egg-free Psyllium Husk Chaffles

Servings: 1

Cooking Time:

4 Minutes

Ingredients:

- 1 ounce Mozzarella cheese, shredded
- 1 tablespoon cream cheese, softened
- 1 tablespoon psyllium husk powder

Directions:

1. Preheat a waffle iron and then grease it.
2. In a blender, place all ingredients and pulse until a slightly crumbly mixture forms.
3. Place the mixture into preheated waffle iron and cook for about 4 minutes or until golden brown.
4. Serve warm.

Nutrition: Calories: 137 Carb: 1.3g Fat: 8.8g Saturated Fat: 2g Carbohydrates: 1.3g Dietary Fiber: 0g Sugar: 0g Protein: 9.5g

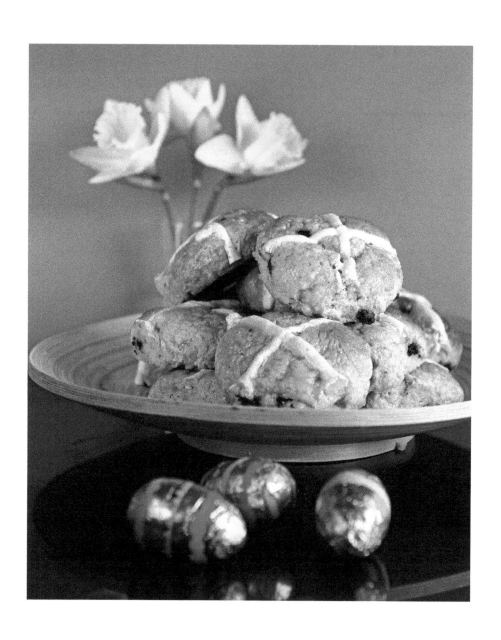

Mozzarella & Almond Flour Chaffles

Servings: 2
Cooking Time:
8 Minutes

Ingredients:

- ½ cup Mozzarella cheese, shredded
- 1 large organic egg
- 2 tablespoons blanched almond flour
- ¼ teaspoon organic baking powder

Directions:

1. Preheat a mini waffle iron and then grease it.
2. In a medium bowl, place all ingredients and with a fork, mix until well combined.
3. Place half of the mixture into preheated waffle iron and cook for about 4 minutes or until golden brown.
4. Repeat with the remaining mixture.
5. Serve warm.

Nutrition: Calories: 98 Net Carb: 1.4g Fat: 7.1g Saturated Fat: 1g Carbohydrates: 2.2g Dietary Fiber: 0.8g Sugar: 0.2g Protein: 7g

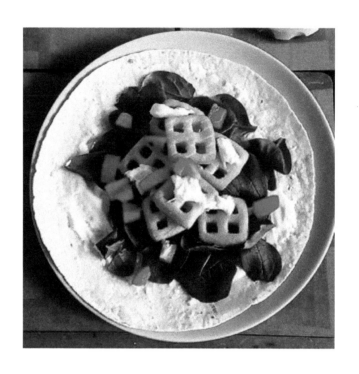

Pulled Pork Chaffle Sandwiches

Servings: 4

Cooking Time:

28 Minutes

Ingredients:

- 2 eggs, beaten
- 1 cup finely grated cheddar cheese
- ¼ tsp baking powder
- 2 cups cooked and shredded pork
- 1 tbsp sugar-free BBQ sauce
- 2 cups shredded coleslaw mix
- 2 tbsp apple cider vinegar
- ½ tsp salt
- ¼ cup ranch dressing

Directions:

1. Preheat the waffle iron.
2. In a medium bowl, mix the eggs, cheddar cheese, and baking powder.
3. Open the iron and add a quarter of the mixture. Close and cook until crispy, 7 minutes.
4. Transfer the chaffle to a plate and make 3 more chaffles in the same manner.
5. Meanwhile, in another medium bowl, mix the pulled pork with the BBQ sauce until well combined. Set aside.
6. Also, mix the coleslaw mix, apple cider vinegar, salt, and ranch dressing in another medium bowl.
7. When the chaffles are ready, on two pieces, divide the pork and then top with the ranch

coleslaw. Cover with the remaining chaffles and insert mini skewers to secure the sandwiches.
8. Enjoy afterward.

Nutrition: Calories: 374 Fats: 23.61g Carbs: 8.2g Protein: 28.05g

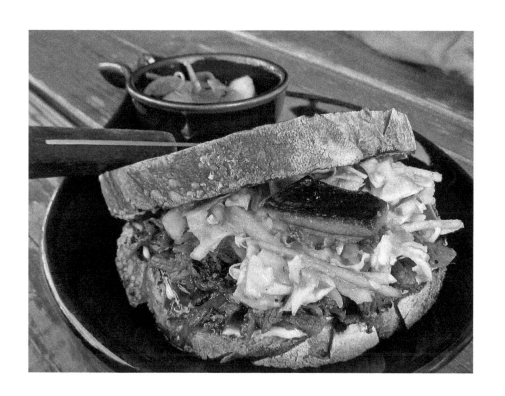

Cheddar & Egg White Chaffles

Servings: 4
Cooking Time:
12 Minutes

Ingredients:

- 2 egg whites
- 1 cup Cheddar cheese, shredded

Directions:

1. Preheat a mini waffle iron and then grease it.
2. In a small bowl, place the egg whites and cheese and stir to combine.
3. Place ¼ of the mixture into preheated waffle iron and cook for about 4 minutes or until golden brown.
4. Repeat with the remaining mixture.
5. Serve warm.

Nutrition: Calories: 122 Carb: 0.5g Fat: 9.4g Saturated Carbohydrates: 0.5g Fiber: 0g Sugar: 0.3g Protein: 8.8g

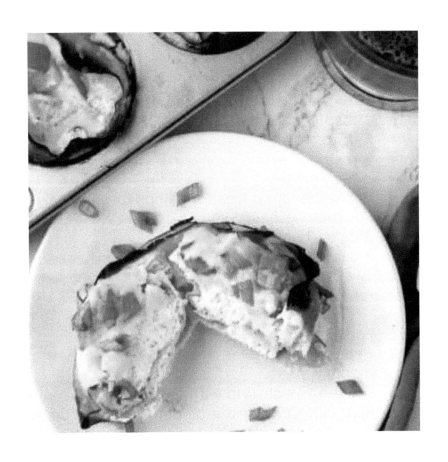

Spicy Shrimp And Chaffles

Servings: 4

Cooking Time:

31 Minutes

Ingredients:

- For the shrimp:
- 1 tbsp olive oil
- 1 lb jumbo shrimp, peeled and deveined
- 1 tbsp Creole seasoning
- Salt to taste
- 2 tbsp hot sauce
- 3 tbsp butter
- 2 tbsp chopped fresh scallions to garnish
- For the chaffles:
- 2 eggs, beaten
- 1 cup finely grated Monterey Jack cheese

Directions:

1. For the shrimp:
2. Heat the olive oil in a medium skillet over medium heat.
3. Season the shrimp with the Creole seasoning and salt. Cook in the oil until pink and opaque on both sides, 2 minutes.
4. Pour in the hot sauce and butter. Mix well until the shrimp is adequately coated in the sauce, 1 minute.
5. Turn the heat off and set aside.
6. For the chaffles:
7. Preheat the waffle iron.
8. In a medium bowl, mix the eggs and Monterey Jack cheese.

9. Open the iron and add a quarter of the mixture. Close and cook until crispy, 7 minutes.
10. Transfer the chaffle to a plate and make 3 more chaffles in the same manner.
11. Cut the chaffles into quarters and place on a plate.
12. Top with the shrimp and garnish with the scallions.
13. Serve warm.

Nutrition: Calories 342 Fats 19.75g Carbs 2.8g Carbs 2.3g Protein 36.01g

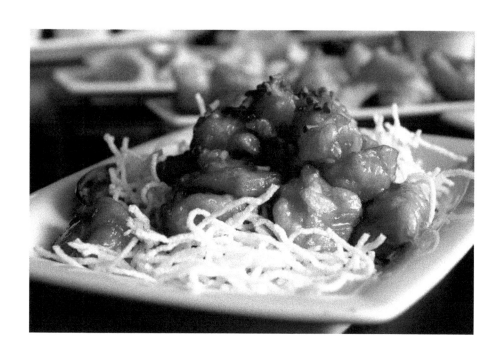

Creamy Chicken Chaffle Sandwich

Servings: 2

Cooking Time:

10 Minutes

Ingredients:

- Cooking spray
- 1 cup chicken breast fillet, cubed
- Salt and pepper to taste
- ¼ cup all-purpose cream
- 4 garlic chaffles
- Parsley, chopped

Directions:

1. Spray your pan with oil.
2. Put it over medium heat.
3. Add the chicken fillet cubes.
4. Season with salt and pepper.
5. Reduce heat and add the cream.
6. Spread chicken mixture on top of the chaffle.
7. Garnish with parsley and top with another chaffle.

Nutrition: Calories 273Total Fat 34g Saturated Fat 4.1g Cholesterol 62mg Sodium 373mg Total Carbohydrate 22.5g Dietary Fiber 1.1g Total Sugars 3.2g Protein 17.5g Potassium 177mg

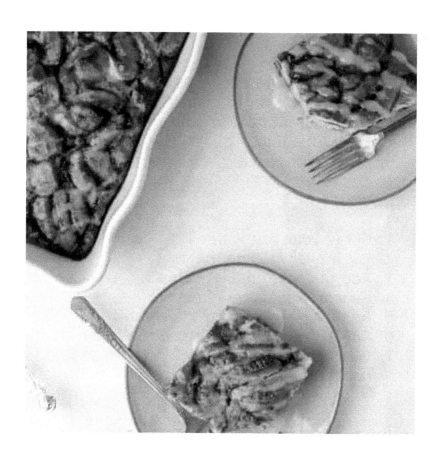

Chaffle Cannoli

Servings: 4

Cooking Time:

28 Minutes

Ingredients:

- For the chaffles:
- 1 large egg
- 1 egg yolk
- 3 tbsp butter, melted
- 1 tbso swerve confectioner's
- 1 cup finely grated Parmesan cheese
- 2 tbsp finely grated mozzarella cheese
- For the cannoli filling:
- ½ cup ricotta cheese
- 2 tbsp swerve confectioner's sugar
- 1 tsp vanilla extract
- 2 tbsp unsweetened chocolate chips for garnishing

Directions:

1. Preheat the waffle iron.
2. Meanwhile, in a medium bowl, mix all the ingredients for the chaffles.
3. Open the iron, pour in a quarter of the mixture, cover, and cook until crispy, 7 minutes.
4. Remove the chaffle onto a plate and make 3 more with the remaining batter.
5. Meanwhile, for the cannoli filling:
6. Beat the ricotta cheese and swerve confectioner's sugar until smooth. Mix in the vanilla.

7. On each chaffle, spread some of the filling and wrap over.
8. Garnish the creamy ends with some chocolate chips.
9. Serve immediately.

Nutrition: Calories 308Fats 25.05gCarbs 5.17gNet Carbs 5.17gProtein 15.18g

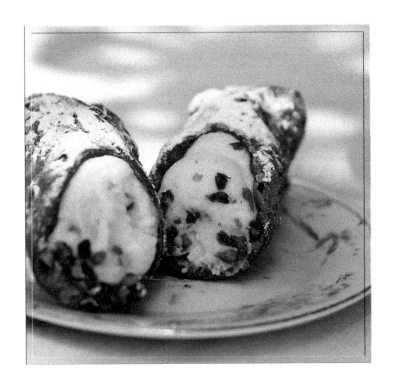

Strawberry Shortcake Chaffle Bowls

Servings: 4

Cooking Time:

28 Minutes

Ingredients:

- 1 egg, beaten
- ½ cup finely grated mozzarella cheese
- 1 tbsp almond flour
- ¼ tsp baking powder
- 2 drops cake batter extract
- 1 cup cream cheese, softened
- 1 cup fresh strawberries, sliced
- 1 tbsp sugar-free maple syrup

Directions:

1. Preheat a waffle bowl maker and grease lightly with cooking spray.
2. Meanwhile, in a medium bowl, whisk all the ingredients except the cream cheese and strawberries.
3. Open the iron, pour in half of the mixture, cover, and cook until crispy, 6 to 7 minutes.
4. Remove the chaffle bowl onto a plate and set aside.
5. Make a second chaffle bowl with the remaining batter.
6. To serve, divide the cream cheese into the chaffle bowls and top with the strawberries.
7. Drizzle the filling with the maple syrup and serve.

Nutrition: Calories 235Fats 20.62gCarbs 5.9g Carbs 5gProtein 7.51g

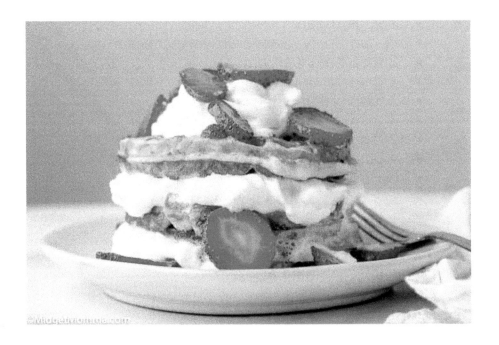

Chocolate Melt Chaffles

Servings: 4

Cooking Time:

36 Minutes

Ingredients:

- For the chaffles:
- 2 eggs, beaten
- ¼ cup finely grated Gruyere cheese
- 2 tbsp heavy cream
- 1 tbsp coconut flour
- 2 tbsp cream cheese, softened
- 3 tbsp unsweetened cocoa powder
- 2 tsp vanilla extract
- A pinch of salt
- For the chocolate sauce:
- 1/3 cup + 1 tbsp heavy cream
- 1 ½ oz unsweetened baking chocolate, chopped
- 1 ½ tsp sugar-free maple syrup
- 1 ½ tsp vanilla extract

Directions:

1. For the chaffles:
2. Preheat the waffle iron.
3. In a medium bowl, mix all the ingredients for the chaffles.
4. Open the iron and add a quarter of the mixture. Close and cook until crispy, 7 minutes.
5. Transfer the chaffle to a plate and make 3 more with the remaining batter.
6. For the chocolate sauce:

7. Pour the heavy cream into saucepan and simmer over low heat, 3 minutes.
8. Turn the heat off and add the chocolate. Allow melting for a few minutes and stir until fully melted, 5 minutes.
9. Mix in the maple syrup and vanilla extract.
10. Assemble the chaffles in layers with the chocolate sauce sandwiched between each layer.
11. Slice and serve immediately.

Nutrition: Calories 172Fats 13.57gCarbs 6.65gNet Carbs 3.65gProtein 5.76g

Pumpkin & Pecan Chaffle

Servings: 2

Cooking Time:

10 Minutes

Ingredients:

- 1 egg, beaten
- ½ cup mozzarella cheese, grated
- ½ teaspoon pumpkin spice
- 1 tablespoon pureed pumpkin
- 2 tablespoons almond flour
- 1 teaspoon sweetener
- 2 tablespoons pecans, chopped

Directions:

1. Turn on the waffle maker.
2. Beat the egg in a bowl.
3. Stir in the rest of the ingredients.
4. Pour half of the mixture into the device.
5. Seal the lid.
6. Cook for 5 minutes.
7. Remove the chaffle carefully.
8. Repeat the steps to make the second chaffle.

Nutrition: Calories 210Total Fat 17 g Saturated Fat 10 g Cholesterol 110 mg Sodium 250 mg Potassium 570 Total Carbohydrate 4.6 g Dietary Fiber 1.7 g Protein 11 g Total Sugars 2 g

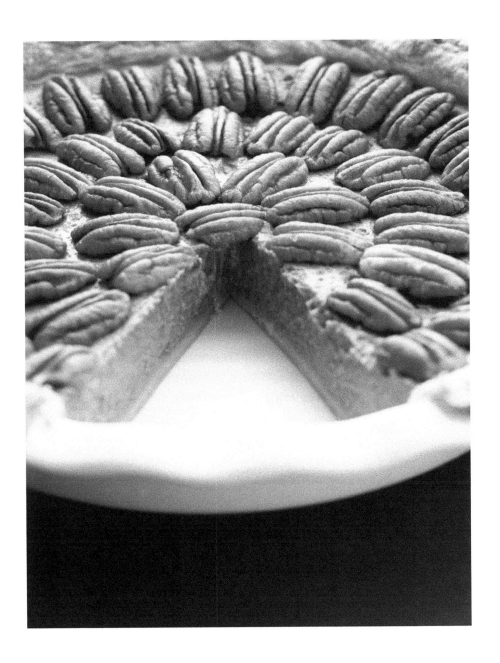

Spicy Jalapeno & Bacon Chaffles

Servings:2

Cooking Time:

5 Minutes

Ingredients:

- 1 oz. cream cheese
- 1 large egg
- 1/2 cup cheddar cheese
- 2 tbsps. bacon bits
- 1/2 tbsp. jalapenos
- 1/4 tsp baking powder

Directions:

1. Switch on your waffle maker.
2. Grease your waffle maker with cooking spray and let it heat up.
3. Mix together egg and vanilla extract in a bowl first.
4. Add baking powder, jalapenos and bacon bites.
5. Add in cheese last and mix together.
6. Pour the chaffles batter intothe maker and cook the chaffles for about 2-3 minutesutes.
7. Once chaffles are cooked, remove from the maker.
8. Serve hot and enjoy!

Nutrition: Protein: 24% 5kcal Fat: 70% 175 kcal
Carbohydrates: 6% 15 kcal

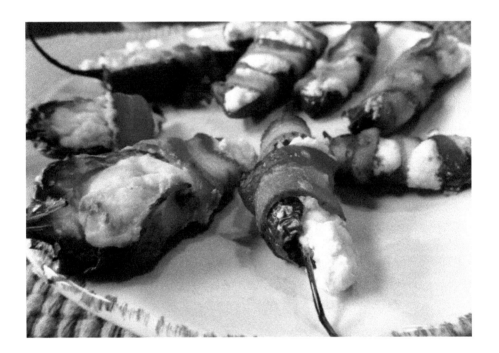

Zucchini Parmesan Chaffles

Servings: 2

Cooking Time:

14 Minutes

Ingredients:

- 1 cup shredded zucchini
- 1 egg, beaten
- ½ cup finely grated Parmesan cheese
- Salt and freshly ground black pepper to taste

Directions:

1. Preheat the waffle iron.
2. Put all the ingredients in a medium bowl and mix well.
3. Open the iron and add half of the mixture. Close and cook until crispy, 7 minutes.
4. Remove the chaffle onto a plate and make another with the remaining mixture.
5. Cut each chaffle into wedges and serve afterward.

Nutrition: Calories 138Fats 9.07gCarbs 3.81gNet Carbs 3.71gProtein 10.02g

Cheddar & Almond Flour Chaffles

Servings: 2

Cooking Time:

10 Minutes

Ingredients:

- 1 large organic egg, beaten
- ½ cup Cheddar cheese, shredded
- 2 tablespoons almond flour

Directions:

1. Preheat a mini waffle iron and then grease it.
2. In a bowl, place the egg, Cheddar cheese and almond flour and beat until well combined.
3. Place half of the mixture into preheated waffle iron and cook for about 5 minutes or until golden brown.
4. Repeat with the remaining mixture.
5. Serve warm.

Nutrition: Calories: 195Net Carb: 1gFat: 15.Saturated Fat: 7gCarbohydrates: 1.8gDietary Fiber: 0.8g Sugar: 0.6gProtein: 10.2g

Simple& Beginner Chaffle

Servings:2
Cooking Time:
5 Minutes

Ingredients:

- 1 large egg
- 1/2 cup mozzarella cheese, shredded
- Cooking spray

Directions:

1. Switch on your waffle maker.
2. Beat the egg with a fork in a small mixing bowl.
3. Once the egg is beaten, add the mozzarella and mix well.
4. Spray the waffle makerwith cooking spray.
5. Pour the chaffles mixture in a preheated waffle maker and let it cook for about 2-3 minutes.
6. Once the chaffles are cooked, carefully remove them from the maker and cook the remaining batter.
7. Serve hot with coffee and enjoy!

Nutrition: Protein: 36% 42 kcal Fat: 60% 71 kcal Carbohydrates: 4% 5 kcal

Asian Cauliflower Chaffles

Servings: 4

Cooking Time:

28 Minutes

Ingredients:

- For the chaffles:
- 1 cup cauliflower rice, steamed
- 1 large egg, beaten
- Salt and freshly ground black pepper to taste
- 1 cup finely grated Parmesan cheese
- 1 tsp sesame seeds
- ¼ cup chopped fresh scallions
- For the dipping sauce:
- 3 tbsp coconut aminos
- 1 ½ tbsp plain vinegar
- 1 tsp fresh ginger puree
- 1 tsp fresh garlic paste
- 3 tbsp sesame oil
- 1 tsp fish sauce
- 1 tsp red chili flakes

Directions:

1. Preheat the waffle iron.
2. In a medium bowl, mix the cauliflower rice, egg, salt, black pepper, and Parmesan cheese.
3. Open the iron and add a quarter of the mixture. Close and cook until crispy, 7 minutes.
4. Transfer the chaffle to a plate and make 3 more chaffles in the same manner.
5. Meanwhile, make the dipping sauce.

6. In a medium bowl, mix all the ingredients for the dipping sauce.
7. Plate the chaffles, garnish with the sesame seeds and scallions and serve with the dipping sauce.

Nutrition: Calories 231 Fats 188g Carbs 5.42g Protein 9.66g

Sharp Cheddar Chaffles

Servings: 2

Cooking Time:

10 Minutes

Ingredients:

- 1 organic egg, beaten
- ½ cup sharp Cheddar cheese, shredded

Directions:

1. Preheat a mini waffle iron and then grease it.
2. In a small bowl, place the egg and cheese and stir to combine.
3. Place half of the mixture into preheated waffle iron and cook for about 5 minutes or until golden brown.
4. Repeat with the remaining mixture.
5. Serve warm.

Nutrition: Calories: 145Net Carb: 0.5g Fat: 11 Saturated Fat: 6.6 g Carbohydrates: 0.5g Fiber: 0g Sugar: 0.3g Protein: 9.8g

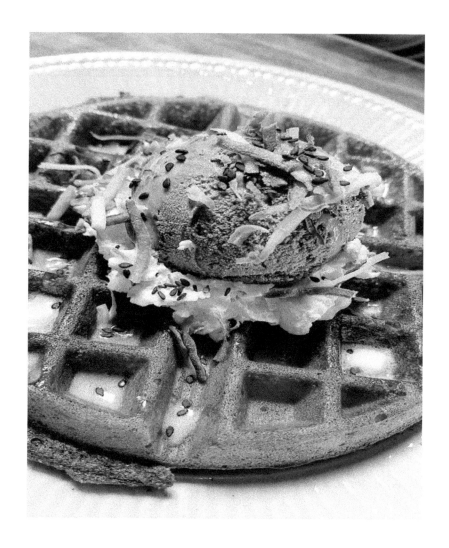

Egg-free Almond Flour Chaffles

Servings: 2

Cooking Time:

10 Minutes

Ingredients:

- 2 tablespoons cream cheese, softened
- 1 cup mozzarella cheese, shredded
- 2 tablespoons almond flour
- 1 teaspoon organic baking powder

Directions:

1. Preheat a mini waffle iron and then grease it.
2. In a medium bowl, place all ingredients and with a fork, mix until well combined.
3. Place half of the mixture into preheated waffle iron and cook for about 4-5 minutes or until golden brown.
4. Repeat with the remaining mixture.
5. Serve warm.

Nutrition: Calories: 77 Carb: 2.4g Fat: 9.8g Saturated Fat: 4g Carbohydrates: 3.2g Dietary Fiber: 0.8g Sugar: 0.3g Protein: 4.8g

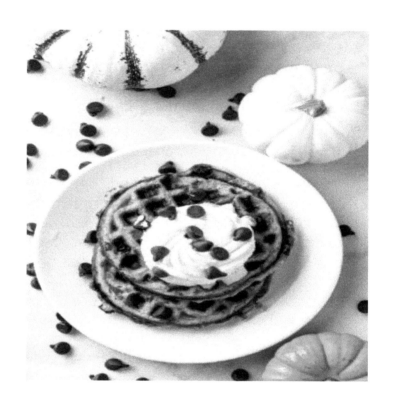

Lightning Source UK Ltd.
Milton Keynes UK
UKHW020730210621
385887UK00005B/135